SURVIVING THE MACHINE

Understanding the Trillion-Dollar Wealth Transfer and the Great Healthcare Purge to Survive 2026 and Beyond

Raymond Fremont

THE FINE PRINT

Maryland, USA

ISBN: 978-1-64973-189-0

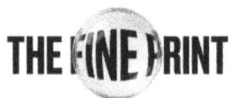

THE FINE PRINT

Each section of the book is followed by citations from the Congressional Research Service (CRS) summaries of H.R. 1, rather than the raw legislative statute. The CRS is a non-partisan research institute within the Library of Congress. Their summaries are widely considered the "gold standard" for understanding legislation because they translate complex statutory language (e.g., "Strike paragraph 3 and insert...") into plain English explanations of the policy's legal effect. These summaries are considered non-partisan by all branches of the government and major political parties in the United States, including Democrats and Republicans. CRS summaries do not add opinions or other extraneous information; they simply convert highly technical jargon into readable, understandable language relied upon by members of Congress from all parties..

LINKS TO FULL TEXTS

Link to H.R. 1: Bill Summary (119th Congress)

https://www.congress.gov/bill/119th-congress/house-bill/1#summary

Link to H.R. 1: Full Bill Text (119th Congress)

https://www.govinfo.gov/app/details/PLAW-119publ21

CONTENTS

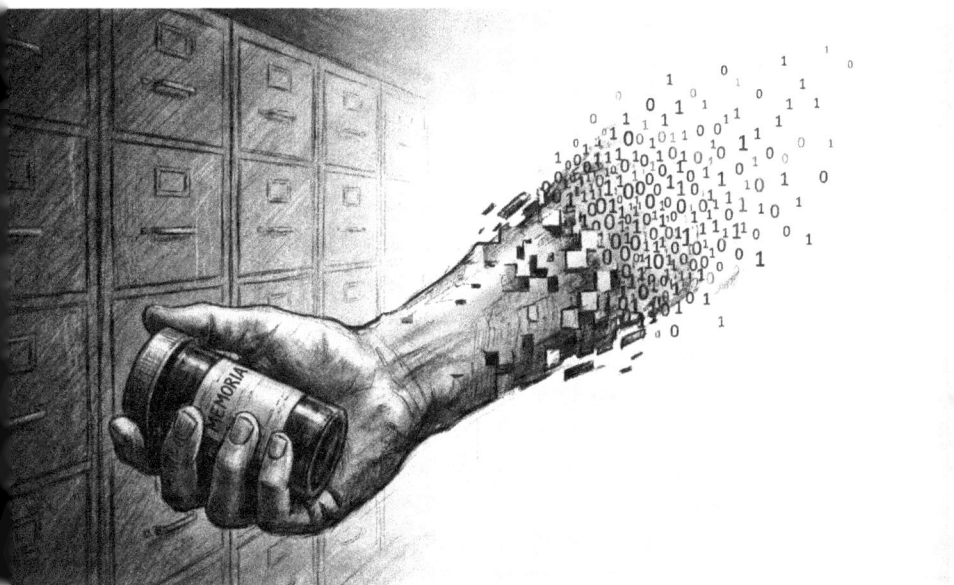

FOREWORD
TEN MILLION GHOSTS

T hey call it the "One Big Beautiful Bill Act". The name is printed right there on page one. It sits under the official stamp of the 119th Congress. The font is serif. Professional. It looks like legislation.

It feels like a trap door.

Politicians love to talk about "slashing" budgets. They use violent verbs. They pretend they are warriors wielding broadswords against the deficit. But that is not how this bill works. There is no sword. There is only a slow, bureaucratic suffocation.

This document is 46 pages of fine print designed to make you disappear.

Read Section 71119. It introduces "Personal Accountability". That sounds nice. Who doesn't want accountability? But look closer. It demands 80 hours of work, community service, or study (in combination) every single month for Medicaid expansion enrollees. Not 79 hours. Eighty. You need to prove it.. You need to verify it.

Miss a shift? You're a ghost. Lose the pay stub? Ghost. The website crashes while you're uploading your community service log? Ghost.

The bill calls this "Increasing Personal Accountability". A behavioral economist calls it a friction cost. It is a hurdle set just high enough to trip the exhausted.

Then there is the silence.

Section 71104 demands a check of the "Death Master File" every quarter. That sounds efficient. We shouldn't pay benefits to the deceased. But databases are messy. People have similar names. Social Security numbers get transposed by a tired data entry clerk in a basement office. When the computer decides you are dead, you stop existing in the system. Your coverage vanishes. You walk into a pharmacy to pick up insulin. The pharmacist shakes his head. The register hums.

You are standing there. Breathing. Alive. But the system sees a ghost.

This act creates millions of them.

It targets the edges. It strips eligibility from "lawfully present" immigrants who have played by the rules. It demands that if you received a dollar too much in tax credits, you pay back every single cent. No cap. No mercy. It freezes the funding for rural hospitals, squeezing the only ER in the county until the lights go out.

The air conditioning in the waiting room stutters. Then it stops.

We are looking at a future where 10 million people vanish from the rolls. They won't die immediately. They will just fade. They will skip the checkup. They will ration the pills. They will wait until the chest pain is unbearable before calling 911.

This book is not about the deficit. The bill claims to save money. It claims to increase the debt limit by $5 trillion. Those are just numbers.

This book is about the friction. It is about the specific, intentional barriers erected between you and your survival. We are going to take this bill apart. We will look at the gears. We will examine the traps.

By the end, you will know exactly how the trick is performed. You will see how the floor drops out.

Welcome to the machine.

CITATIONS

SECTION 71119

"This section requires, beginning not later than the first quarter after December 31, 2026... individuals who are eligible for Medicaid as part of the Medicaid expansion population to engage in community service, work, or other activities... Specifically, the section requires these individuals to, on a monthly basis, (1) work at least 80 hours, (2) complete at least 80 hours of community service..."

SECTION 71104

"This section requires state Medicaid programs to check, beginning in 2028, the SSA's Death Master File on at least a quarterly basis to determine whether Medicaid enrollees are deceased."

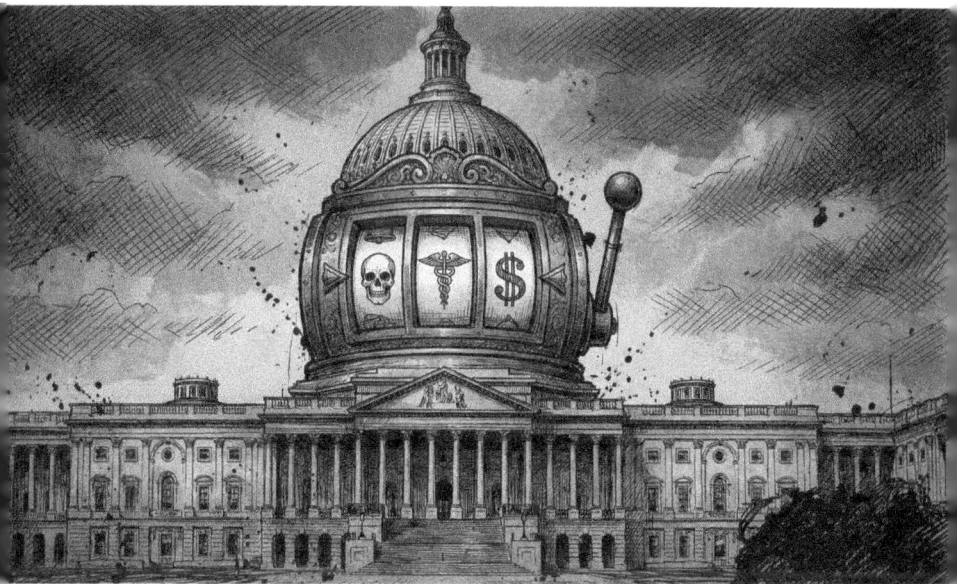

INTRODUCTION:
THE CASINO IS OPEN

The House is betting the farm.

They didn't hide the stakes. Section 72001 puts the number on the board in black and white. Five trillion dollars. That is the new debt limit. That is the buy-in.

Most bills are boring. They fix potholes. They rename post offices. They die in committee.

This bill is different. H.R. 1 is a "reconciliation" bill. That is a technical term for a legislative bulldozer. It means the Senate can't filibuster it. It means they don't need 60 votes. They just need 51.

They got exactly 51.

The margin was razor-thin. Vice President tie-breakers. Midnight sessions. But in a casino, winning by an inch is the same as winning by a mile. The chips are already raked in.

You are the player.

The "One Big Beautiful Bill Act" is not a plan. It is a redistribution of risk. The government is shedding weight. It is cutting the ropes. It calls this "reducing wasteful spending".

Let's look at the winners.

If you make money, you win. The tax cuts from 2017 are now permanent. The top rate stays at 37%. The corporate tax rate stays low. The Estate Tax exemption—the tax on dead millionaires—jumps to $15 million. That is a jackpot.

If you drill for oil, you win. The royalty rates are slashed. The restrictions on the Arctic National Wildlife Refuge are gone. They are selling leases in the Gulf of Mexico like they are going out of style.

Now look at the losers.

The losers are the people who need a safety net. Section 10101 freezes the cost of the "Thrifty Food Plan". That is the math formula that decides if you eat. It stops accounting for the real cost of a healthy diet. It just tracks inflation.

Real food prices go up. Your benefits stay flat. You eat less.

The losers are the sick. Section 71201 kicks non-citizens off Medicare. Not illegal immigrants. Lawful permanent residents. People who paid taxes. The bill gives the Social Security Administration 18 months to hunt them down and terminate them.

The losers are the unemployed. Section 71119 mandates work. If you don't clock 80 hours a month, you lose your Medicaid.

The casino is efficient.

They call it "Beautiful". The text says "An act to provide for reconciliation". But read the summaries. Read the fine print.

It is a transfer of wealth. It takes stability from the poor and gives liquidity to the rich. It takes food from a hungry child and gives a tax deduction to a corporate jet.

The wheel is spinning. The ball is bouncing.

You didn't ask to play. You didn't sit at the table. But your chips are in the pot.

We are going to walk the floor. We are going to look at every game. We are going to see how the odds are stacked.

First stop: The Great Purge.

CITATIONS

SECTION 72001

"This section increases the statutory debt limit by $5 trillion."

SECTION 10101

"This section prohibits USDA from increasing the cost of the Thrifty Food Plan (TFP) based on a reevaluation of the contents of the TFP... any annual adjustment to the cost of the plan must be based on the Consumer Price Index for All Urban Consumers."

SECTION 71201

"This section generally restricts Medicare eligibility to U.S. citizens, lawful permanent residents, Cuban-Haitian entrants, and Compact of Free Association migrants... The SSA must identify Medicare enrollees who do not meet these requirements and terminate their enrollment within 18 months..."

SECTION 71119

"This section requires... individuals who are eligible for Medicaid as part of the Medicaid expansion population to engage in community service, work, or other activities in order to qualify for Medicaid."

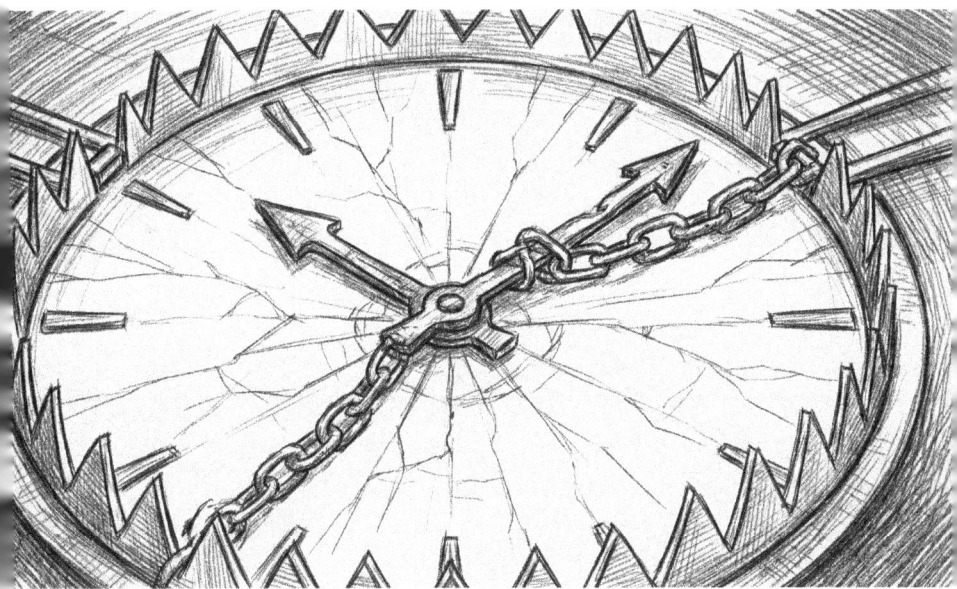

THE EIGHTY-HOUR TRAP

Poverty is a full-time job.

You wait for the bus. You wait at the laundromat. You wait on hold with the utility company.

Now, you have a new boss.

Section 71119 of H.R. 1 isn't asking for much. It just wants 80 hours of your time. Every month. Rain or shine.

If you want to keep your Medicaid, you have to work. Or volunteer. Or study.

Here is the math. 80 hours is a half-time job. 20 hours a week. That sounds reasonable to a Senator. Senators have salaries. They have schedules. They have aides who manage their calendars.

The working poor do not have schedules. They have chaos.

If you are a waiter, your hours depend on the dinner rush. If you are a landscape laborer, your hours depend on the rain. If you drive for Uber, your hours depend on the algorithm.

One week you get 30 hours. The next week you get 10.

If you hit 79 hours in February? You are out. The trap snaps shut.

The bill calls this "Increasing Personal Accountability". It requires able-bodied adults in the expansion population to verify their compliance.

But here is the jagged edge.

It's not just about doing the work. It's about proving it.

You need to submit paperwork. You need a signature from the soup kitchen director where you volunteered. You need pay stubs from the three different apps you drive for.

Section 71119 says you must demonstrate compliance "on a monthly basis".

Imagine the bureaucracy. Millions of people uploading millions of PDF files every thirty days. State servers smoking under the load. A case worker with a stack of files four feet high.

One lost file. One rejected screenshot. One glitch.

You are purged.

The bill offers a "grace period" for new applicants. It is a cruel joke. If you are applying for the first time, you must prove you complied for *one to three months* consecutively *before* you even file the application.

Think about that.

You just lost your job. You are broke. You need health insurance today because your kid has a fever.

The state says: "Come back in ninety days. After you've done your community service."

This isn't a safety net. It is a waiting room with no chairs.

There are exemptions. If you have a child under 13, you are safe. If you have a "serious medical condition," you are safe. But who defines "serious"?

The state does.

If your back hurts so bad you can't stand, but you aren't "disabled" by the Social Security definition, you work. You grind through the pain.

The Congressional Budget Office knows what happens next. They don't call it "laziness." They call it "churn."

People fall off the rolls not because they don't work, but be-

THE BIG BOLD BEAUTIFUL BILL AND YOUR HEALTH

cause they can't navigate the maze. They miss a deadline. They don't understand the form.

The government saves money. The bill allocates $200 million just to build the systems to track this. That is $200 million spent on digital handcuffs.

The savings don't come from people getting jobs. The savings come from people giving up.

It is a war of attrition.

Section 71119 is the siege engine. It starves the beast by starving the patient.

And once you are off the list? Getting back on is harder than ever.

The door is locked. You are outside. And it is starting to rain.

CITATIONS

SECTION 71119

"States must verify an individual's compliance upon a determination or redetermination of eligibility but may also choose to verify compliance more frequently. States may not waive the new requirements."

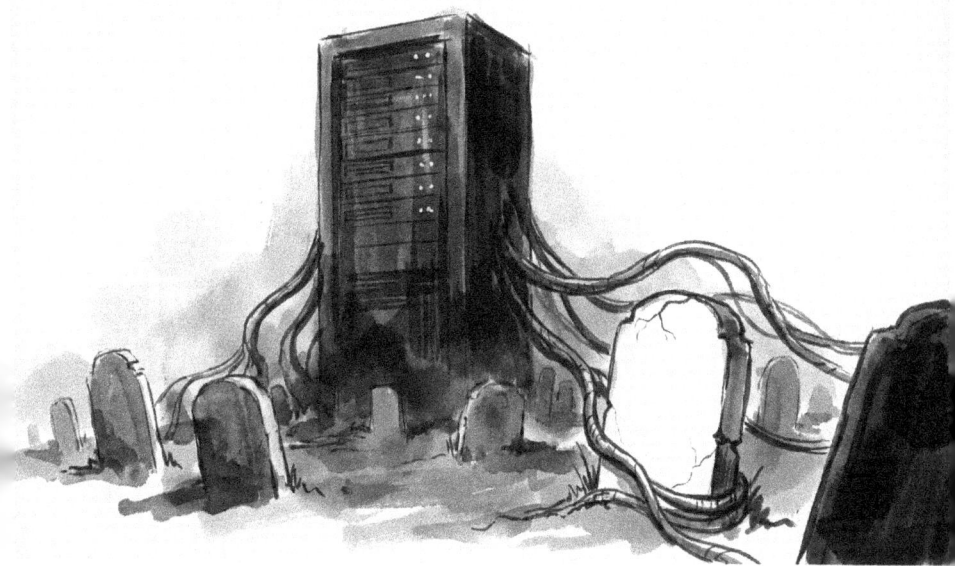

DEATH BY DATABASE

The computer is always right.

That is the premise of modern bureaucracy. If the screen says "Active," you are safe. If the screen says "Ineligible," you are cast out.

H.R. 1 turns the computer into a weapon.

It starts with a list. Section 71104 requires state Medicaid programs to query the Social Security Administration's "Death Master File". They must do this every quarter.

The name sounds like science fiction. The reality is mundane data entry.

The government wants to stop paying for ghosts. That makes sense. We shouldn't send checks to the deceased.

But databases are dirty. They are filled with typos. They are riddled with transposed digits.

If a clerk hits a 5 instead of a 6, you are dead.

The system will flag you. The check will stop. You will go to the doctor for a refill on your heart medication. The claim will be denied.

"The system says you are deceased," the pharmacist will say.

You will argue. You will show your ID. It won't matter. The pharmacist cannot override the Master File. You have to go to the Social Security office. You have to prove you are breathing.

While you fight the zombie tag, you have no coverage.

But being "dead" is rare. The real killer is Section 71107.

This section attacks your time.

Right now, most states check your eligibility once a year. It is an annual ritual. You gather your pay stubs. You survive for another twelve months.

Section 71107 changes the rhythm. It mandates redeterminations every six months for the expansion population.

They doubled the paperwork.

They doubled the friction.

Every six months, you have to prove you are poor enough. Every six months, you have to prove you are working enough.

This is a specific strategy known as "frequency fatigue."

You might pass the first check. You might pass the second. But eventually, you will miss a piece of mail. You will move apartments and forget to update your address. The letter demanding proof of income will go to your old mailbox.

You won't answer. The state will assume you are ineligible. You are purged.

Then there is the trap door behind you.

Life is messy. Accidents happen before you fill out forms.

Under current law, Medicaid offers retroactive coverage. If you get hit by a bus in January, but you are in a coma and don't apply until April, Medicaid covers you for the three months prior. It prevents bankruptcy.

Section 71112 guts this protection.

For the expansion population, retroactive coverage is slashed to one month.

If you crash your car on February 1st and don't get your paperwork submitted until April 1st, you are liable for February.

The hospital bill for that first month is yours. The ambulance ride. The surgery. The ICU stay.

You are poor enough for Medicaid. You are eligible. But because you didn't file the form fast enough—perhaps because you were unconscious—you are now bankrupt.

This is not about fraud.

Section 71103 builds a "centralized system" to track if you are enrolled in two states at once. It sounds like efficiency. It acts like a surveillance net.

States must report your Social Security number monthly. They must track your address.

The goal is to find a reason to say "No."

Did you move across the border to find work? Flagged. Did you forget to close your case in Ohio before opening one in Kentucky? Flagged.

The bill allocates millions of dollars to build these systems. It spends tax money to hire digital bouncers.

They aren't looking for criminals. They are looking for typos.

The result is a system that demands perfection from people who are living in crisis. It demands that you never move. It demands that you never miss a letter. It demands that you stay alive in the database, even if the data entry clerk killed you.

The database is hungry.

And it is about to get fed.

CITATIONS

SECTION 71104

"This section requires state Medicaid programs to check, beginning in 2028, the SSA's Death Master File on at least a quarterly basis..."

SECTION 71107

"This section requires state Medicaid programs to redetermine every six months... the eligibility of individuals who are enrolled in Medicaid as part of the Medicaid expansion population..."

SECTION 71112

"This section shortens the window for retroactive Medicaid coverage. Specifically... for individuals in the Medicaid expansion population, one month prior to the application filing date..."

SECTION 71103

"This section requires the CMS to establish a centralized system for states to check whether enrollees are simultaneously enrolled in Medicaid or the Children's Health Insurance Program (CHIP) in multiple states."

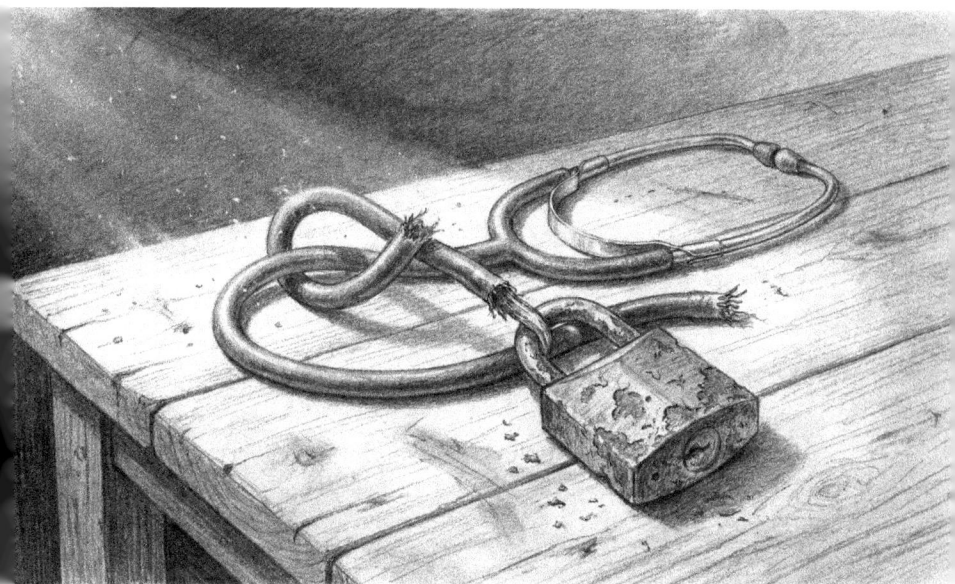

LIGHTS OUT IN THE HEARTLAND

A rural hospital does not die loudly.

There is no explosion. There is no dramatic final ambulance ride.

The death happens in the accounting department.

First, the obstetrics unit closes. Then the MRI machine breaks and nobody fixes it. Then the night shift disappears.

Finally, a padlock goes on the front door. The nearest emergency room is now forty-five miles away. If you have a heart attack, you drive. If you don't make it, you don't make it.

H.R. 1 accelerates this decay.

It targets the financial plumbing that keeps these places alive. It is technical. It is boring. It is lethal.

Turn to Section 71115. The title is "Stopping Abusive Financing Practices". That is political speak for cutting the lifeline.

Here is how the game works today. States want more federal Medicaid money. So they tax their own hospitals. They take that tax revenue and use it to draw down a "match" from the federal government. Then they pay the hospitals back with interest.

It is a gimmick. It is a loophole. But it keeps the lights on in Kentucky and West Virginia.

Section 71115 kills the gimmick.

It freezes the provider tax rate. If a state hasn't expanded Medicaid, it can't raise the tax to get more federal cash. If a state *has* expanded, the allowable tax rate drops. It slides down to 3.5% by 2032.

The flow of easy federal money stops.

The state budget gets a hole in it. The state legislature has two choices. Raise income taxes. Or cut payments to hospitals.

They will cut the payments.

The rural clinic operates on a margin of zero. A 2% cut is not an inconvenience. It is a death sentence.

The bill authors know this. They built a consolation prize.

Section 71401 creates the "Rural Health Transformation Program". It offers $10 billion a year.

That sounds generous.

But look at the mechanism. It is not guaranteed funding. It is an application process.

States must submit "detailed rural health transformation plans". They have to hire consultants to write fifty-page proposals. They have to beg CMS for a slice of the pie.

The money doesn't go to keeping the ER open. It goes to "strategic partnerships" and "workforce training".

You cannot treat a stroke with a strategic partnership.

Then there is the culture war.

Section 71113 targets "Essential Community Providers". These are the clinics that serve the poorest of the poor.

The bill prohibits federal payments to any nonprofit provider that "primarily furnishes family planning services" and offers abortions.

The exceptions are narrow. Rape. Incest. Life of the mother.

If a rural clinic performs a standard abortion, it loses its Medicaid funding for everything. It loses money for diabetes screenings. It loses money for flu shots.

In a city, you can go to a different clinic. In a rural county, there is often only one clinic.

If you defund it, you create a medical desert.

Section 71116 tightens the screws on the big guys too. It limits payments to academic medical centers. These are the big city hospitals where rural patients get airlifted for trauma.

The bill caps their Medicaid payments at the Medicare rate.

Hospitals lose money on Medicare rates. They rely on commercial insurance to subsidize the loss. This bill removes the subsidy.

The ecosystem collapses.

The small rural hospital closes because the provider tax vanished. The local clinic closes because it got defunded for providing reproductive care. The big trauma center stops accepting transfers because it can't afford the overhead.

You are left with a map full of holes.

This is not an accident. It is a controlled demolition of the safety net in the places that need it most.

The bill calls it "transformation."

The transformation is simple. The hospital becomes a Spirit Halloween store.

And you become a statistic.

CITATIONS

SECTION 71115

"The section precludes states that have not expanded Medicaid from increasing the rate of a provider tax beyond that currently in effect... For states that have expanded Medicaid... the maximum rate gradually decreases... with a maximum rate of 3.5% beginning in FY2032..."

SECTION 71401

"States must submit detailed rural health transformation plans and certify that no funds will be used to finance the non-federal share of Medicaid or CHIP."

SECTION 71113

"This section prohibits federal Medicaid payment for one year to nonprofit health care providers that serve predominantly low-income, medically underserved individuals... if the provider (1) primarily furnishes family planning services..."

SECTION 71116

"limit state-directed payments for... academic medical center under Medicaid managed care contracts to the payment rate for services under Medicare, rather than the average commercial rate."

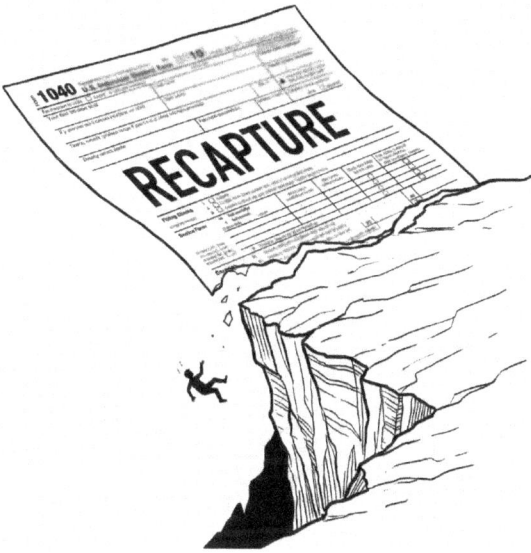

THE SUBSIDY CLIFF

January 1, 2026. Mark the date.

That is when the bill comes due.

For the last few years, the middle class has lived in a bubble. The "enhanced" premium tax credits made health insurance artificially cheap. You went to the exchange. You typed in your income. The silver plan cost you $50 a month.

It felt like a deal.

H.R. 1 pops the bubble.

The bill does not extend those enhanced credits. It lets them die. It lets the price of your premium snap back to reality.

Suddenly, $50 becomes $400.

But high prices are just the start. The real weapon is hidden in the tax code. It is a provision that turns the IRS into a debt collector for the insurance companies.

Turn to Section 71305. The header is "Recapture of Excess Advance Payments".

Here is how the trap works.

You apply for insurance in December. You have to guess your income for the *next* year. You are a freelancer. You drive a truck. You sell houses. You don't know what you will make.

You guess $40,000. The government gives you a tax credit based on that number. They pay the insurer directly.

Then you have a good year. You hustle. You pick up extra shifts. You make $60,000.

Under current law, there is a "safe harbor." The government knows guessing is hard. They cap how much you have to pay back if you were wrong. They limit the damage.

Section 71305 deletes the cap.

It demands "full recapture."

If you underestimated your income, you owe the IRS every single dollar of subsidy you received.

You could owe $6,000. You could owe $10,000.

The bill punishes you for succeeding. It punishes you for not being able to predict the future.

It gets worse.

They don't trust you to tell the truth anymore.

Section 71303 introduces mandatory verification.

Before this bill, the exchanges operated on trust. You attested to your income. You got covered. The IRS checked the math later.

Now, the exchange *must* verify your household income and family size before the credit flows.

You are standing at the pharmacy counter. You need coverage now. But the exchange computer is waiting for a tax transcript from two years ago.

It is the same friction we saw in Medicaid. It is paperwork as a gatekeeper.

Section 71304 tightens the screws on "Special Enrollment Periods."

These are the windows that open when life falls apart. You get divorced. You lose your job. You move.

The bill says you cannot get a premium tax credit during these periods if you are enrolling based on income estimation.

It assumes you are lying. It blocks the exit.

The result is a pincer movement.

On one side, the premiums skyrocket because the subsidies expire. On the other side, the IRS waits with a sledgehammer if you miscalculate your ability to pay.

You are forced to make a bet.

Do you buy the insurance and risk a $10,000 tax bill? Or do you go naked?

Most people will choose the risk. They will buy the plan. They will pray their income stays low.

Then April 15th comes.

The letter arrives.

The cliff is not just a metaphor. It is a line item on your tax return.

And you just fell off.

CITATIONS

SECTION 71305

"This section eliminates the limit on the recapture of excess advance payments of the premium tax credit and, accordingly, allows the full amount of any such excess payments to be recaptured."

SECTION 71303

"This section requires the verification, beginning in 2028, of certain information for an individual to enroll in a health insurance plan through a health insurance exchange... verify... household income and family size, whether the individual is an eligible alien..."

SECTION 71304

"This section provides that the premium tax credit is not allowed for any health insurance plan enrolled in... during a special enrollment period... on the basis of the relationship between the individual's expected household income to the federal poverty level..."

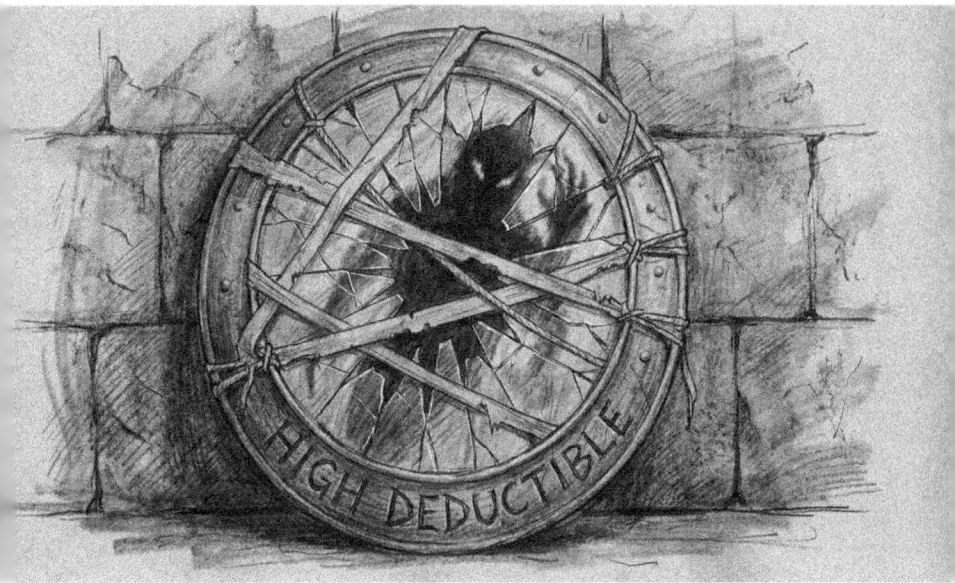
HIGH DEDUCTIBLE

THE BRONZE ILLUSION

The insurance industry loves metals.

Gold. Silver. Bronze.

It sounds like the Olympics. It implies that even if you come in third, you are still a winner.

Section 71307 reveals the truth. Bronze is not a medal. It is a warning label.

For years, the government tried to steer you toward "Silver" plans. These were the middle ground. They had subsidies. They had cost-sharing reductions. They actually paid for things.

H.R. 1 wants you to downgrade.

It unlocks the Health Savings Account (HSA) for the bottom of the barrel.

Previously, to get the tax perks of an HSA, you needed a specific kind of High Deductible Health Plan. It was a strict definition.

Section 71307 kicks the door open. It says you can now pair

an HSA with a "Bronze" plan. Or even a "Catastrophic" plan.

The word "Catastrophic" is doing a lot of heavy lifting.

These plans are designed for the worst day of your life. They are not designed for Tuesday.

If you have a Catastrophic plan, you pay for everything. You pay for the flu shot. You pay for the strep test. You pay for the twisted ankle.

The deductible is a mountain. You have to climb over $9,000 of your own bills before the insurance company spends a dime.

The bill calls this "Enhancing Choice".

Here is the illusion. They tell you that you can save money tax-free in your HSA to pay for that deductible.

But do the math.

To fill an HSA, you need disposable income. You need extra cash at the end of the month.

The people buying Catastrophic plans are usually doing it because they are broke. They are buying the cheapest premium possible because the rent is due.

They don't have $5,000 to park in an investment account.

So they get the high deductible. They get the risk. They get zero tax benefit.

The only people who win are the Healthy Wealthy.

If you are rich and healthy, this is a gift. You buy a cheap Catastrophic plan. You max out your HSA. You invest the money in the stock market tax-free. You treat it like a 401(k) on steroids.

You exit the risk pool.

Section 71308 widens the exit ramp. It allows HSA money to pay for "Direct Primary Care".

This is concierge medicine. You pay a doctor a flat monthly fee—up to $150 a month. You get unlimited visits. No insurance necessary.

It sounds nice. It smells like sterile gauze and old magazines.

But think about the macro effect.

The healthy people leave the standard insurance market. They buy Catastrophic plans and Direct Primary Care. They stop paying premiums into the big pot that covers the sick people.

The risk pool gets sicker.

The premiums for everyone else go up.

It is a death spiral.

The bill encourages this segmentation. It wants the healthy to secede from the sick.

Section 71306 adds "telehealth-only" plans to the mix. You can have an HSA even if your plan essentially just covers a Zoom call with a doctor.

The result is a fractured marketplace.

You will see ads for "affordable" coverage. They will promise low premiums. They will tout the tax advantages.

You will sign up. You will feel responsible.

Then you will get sick. You will go to the specialist. The receptionist will ask for your card.

She will run it. She will look at you.

"You have a $10,000 deductible," she will say. "How would you like to pay?"

The credit card terminal will beep.

That is the sound of the Bronze Illusion shattering.

CITATIONS

SECTION 71307

"This section expands eligibility to make tax-deductible HSA contributions to include individuals who have a bronze-level or catastrophic health insurance plan through a health insurance exchange."

SECTION 71308

"This section expands eligibility to make tax-deductible HSA contributions to include individuals who have a direct primary care service arrangement..."

SECTION 71306

"This section allows individuals to establish and make tax-deductible contributions to a health savings account (HSA) if covered by a health insurance plan that provides telehealth and other remote care services without requiring a deductible..."

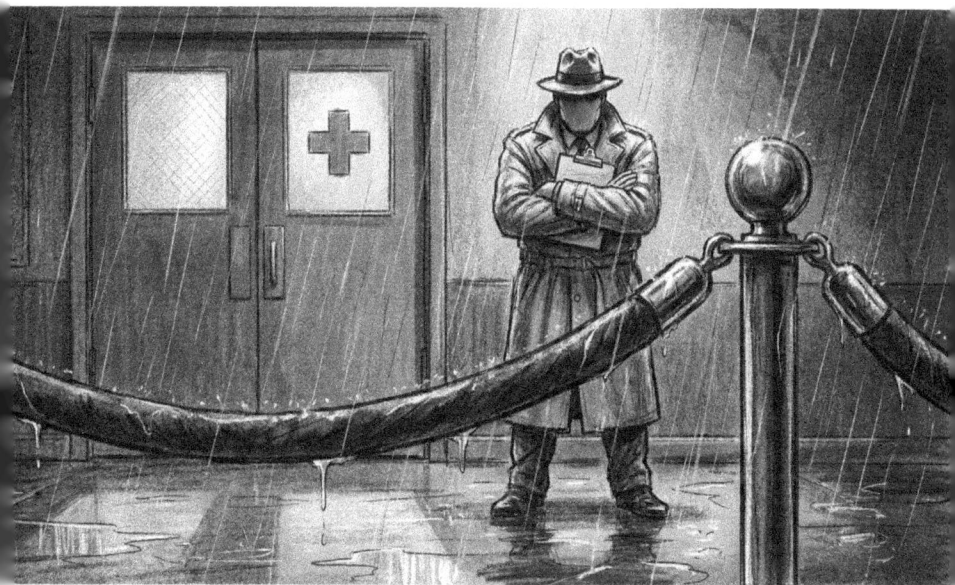

THE VELVET ROPE

Insurance companies used to exclude you for being sick. They called it a "pre-existing condition."

The law banned that. They can't say "No" because you have cancer anymore.

So the strategy changed. Now they just make it impossible to say "Yes."

H.R. 1 erects a velvet rope around the marketplace. It installs a bouncer at the door.

The bouncer's name is Verification.

Turn to Section 71303. It demands the "verification" of your life story before you can buy a plan with a tax credit.

The exchange must verify your household income. It must verify your family size. It must verify your "eligible alien" status. It must verify your place of residence.

This happens *beginning in 2028*.

It sounds responsible. Banks do it. Landlords do it.

But health insurance is not a mortgage. It is an emergency utility.

Under the old rules, the exchange relied on your "attestation." You signed a digital affidavit saying, "I make $30,000." You got your insurance. If you lied, the IRS caught you next April.

Section 71303 kills the honor system. It demands documents upfront.

Imagine the friction.

You are a gig worker. You don't have a W-2. You have a stack of messy 1099s and some Venmo screenshots. The exchange computer says "Upload Proof of Income."

You upload a bank statement. The system rejects it.

You upload a tax return from last year. The system says it's too old.

You call the help line. You wait on hold for three hours.

While you fight the document war, you are uninsured. If you get appendicitis while the "Pending Verification" icon is spinning, you pay the full hospital bill.

The rope stays up.

Then they lock the side doors.

Section 71304 targets "Special Enrollment Periods" (SEPs).

These are the exceptions. The marketplace usually only opens for a few weeks in the fall. SEPs let you in during the rest of the year.

Currently, if your income drops near the poverty line, you can often trigger an SEP. It is a safety valve. If you go broke, you can get covered.

The bill plugs the valve.

It specifically bans premium tax credits for SEPs granted "on the basis of the relationship between the individual's expected household income to the federal poverty level".

Translation: Being poor is no longer a valid excuse to buy insurance late.

You have to wait for a "qualifying life event." Marriage. Birth. Losing other coverage.

Simply running out of money doesn't count.

If you lose your freelance clients in March and your income

crashes, you cannot just sign up for a subsidized plan. You are locked out until November.

You have to survive the spring. You have to survive the summer. You have to survive the autumn.

Hope you don't step on a rusty nail.

The bill even attacks the Tax Credit for your kids.

Section 70104 requires a "work-eligible Social Security number" for every qualifying child.

Previously, certain immigrants could use an ITIN (Individual Taxpayer Identification Number) to claim credits. They paid taxes. They followed the law.

The bill says "Not Today."

No SSN? No credit.

The barrier is not the price. The barrier is the ID card. The barrier is the PDF upload.

This is the new discrimination. They don't ban the sick. They ban the disorganized. They ban the transient. They ban the people who can't produce a "work-eligible" Social Security card on demand.

The marketplace is technically open to everyone.

Just like the Ritz Carlton is open to everyone.

You just have to get past the rope.

CITATIONS

SECTION 71303

"verify... household income and family size, whether the individual is an eligible alien, any health coverage status or eligibility for coverage, place of residence..."

SECTION 71304

"the premium tax credit is not allowed... during a special enrollment period... on the basis of the relationship between the individual's expected household income to the federal poverty level..."

SECTION 70104

"Beginning in 2025, under this section, a taxpayer must provide a work-eligible Social Security number for themselves, for their spouse (if filing jointly), and for each qualifying child."

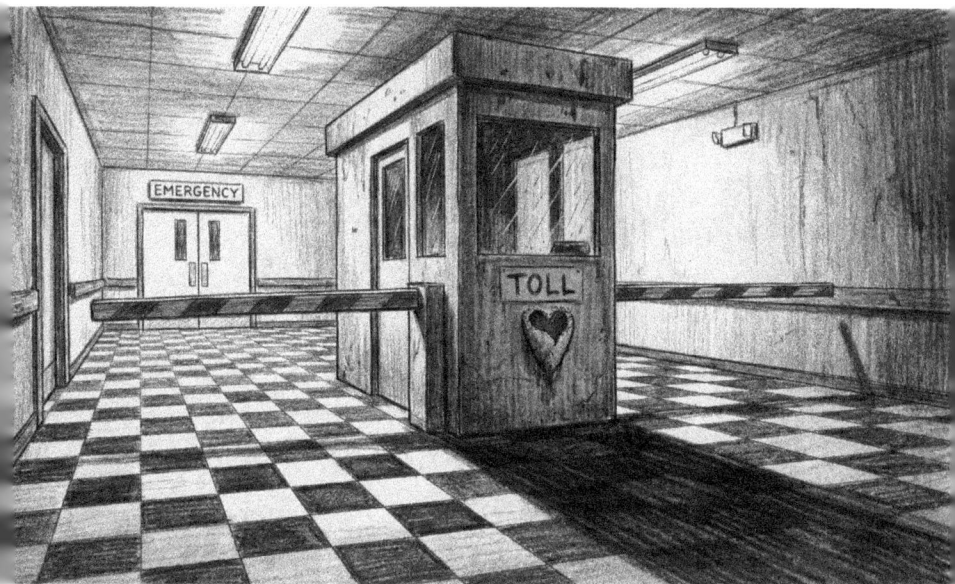

THE ER TAX

You can ban a person from a spreadsheet. You cannot ban them from having a heart attack.

That is the fundamental flaw in H.R. 1's logic on immigration.

The bill tries to solve a financial problem by deleting people.

Turn to Section 71109. It strips Medicaid eligibility from huge swathes of "lawfully residing" immigrants. Refugees. Asylum seekers. People who have papers, but not the *right* papers.

Turn to Section 71201. It does the same for Medicare. It gives the government 18 months to identify and purge these "non-qualified" seniors.

The goal is to save money. If you stop paying for their insulin, the budget looks better.

But biology does not care about your budget.

When you take away the insulin, the diabetic does not disappear. They get sicker. Their blood sugar spikes. They go into ketoacidosis.

Then they collapse.

And where do they go?

They go to the Emergency Room.

Federal law (EMTALA) says the ER *must* stabilize them. They cannot turn them away.

So the ambulance arrives. The doctors work. The ICU bed fills up. The bill runs up to $50,000.

Who pays?

The patient has no insurance. They were kicked off. The hospital tries to bill Medicaid.

But look at Section 71110.

This is the kicker. The bill anticipates this exact scenario. It knows these people will end up in the ER.

So Section 71110 *cuts the reimbursement rate* for emergency services provided to these individuals. It lowers the federal match.

It essentially says to the hospital: "You have to treat them. But we aren't going to pay you the full rate for it."

The hospital is now holding a bag of uncompensated debt.

Hospitals are not charities. They are businesses. When they lose money on the ER, they have to make it up somewhere else.

They raise prices.

A Tylenol becomes $15. An MRI becomes $3,000.

Your insurance company pays the higher rate. Then they raise your premium next year.

This is the "ER Tax."

It is a hidden tax levied on every single American with a health insurance card.

You are paying for the "savings" in H.R. 1. You are paying for the dialysis that happens in the ICU instead of the clinic. You are paying for the emergency surgery that could have been a $20 prescription.

The bill pretends that if you cut coverage, the cost vanishes.

It is a lie.

The cost just migrates. It moves from the efficient line item (preventive care) to the catastrophic line item (emergency care).

And then it lands on your kitchen table in the form of a premium hike.

We are all paying the toll. We just don't see the booth.

CITATIONS

SECTION 71109

"This section generally restricts, beginning in FY2027, federal payment for Medicaid and CHIP to services for individuals who are U.S. residents and are either U.S. citizens, lawful permanent residents, Cuban-Haitian entrants, or Compact of Free Association migrants..."

SECTION 71201

"This section generally restricts Medicare eligibility to U.S. citizens, lawful permanent residents... The SSA must identify Medicare enrollees who do not meet these requirements and terminate their enrollment within 18 months..."

SECTION 71110

"This section reduces the Medicaid federal matching rate for emergency services provided to individuals who are not lawfully residing in the United States... to the same matching rate as would otherwise apply for such services (rather than the enhanced federal matching rate...)."

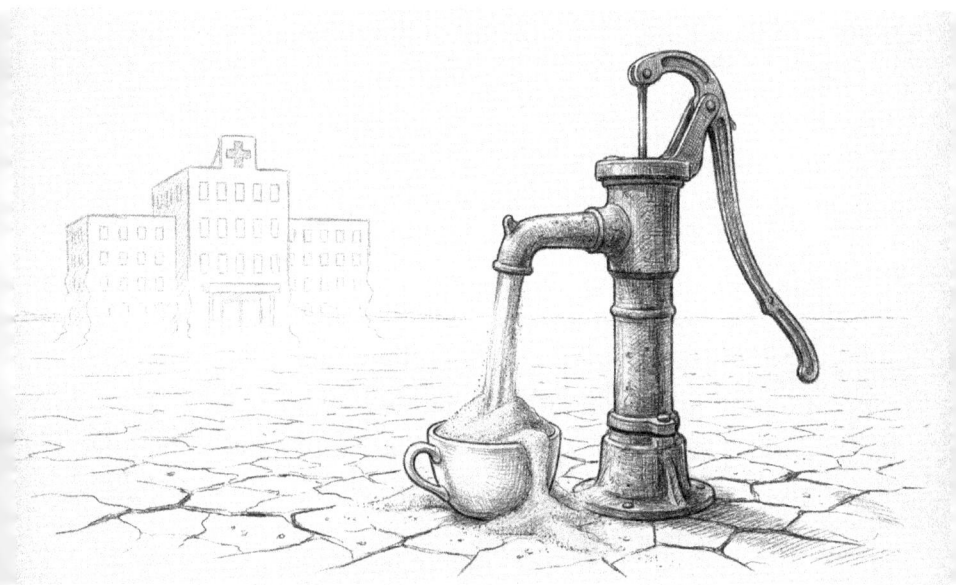

THE MIRAGE OF FUNDING

Politics is the art of giving with one hand while taking with the other.

Usually, the "take" is hidden in the footnotes.

H.R. 1 is bolder. It puts the "take" on the front page and the "give" in a lockbox you can't open.

The problem is undeniable. Rural healthcare is collapsing. Hospitals are closing. Doctors are retiring.

The bill acknowledges this. It offers a solution.

Section 71401 creates the "Rural Health Transformation Program".

It sounds heroic. Transformation. Progress. A bridge to the future.

The price tag is impressive: $10 billion a year for five years. That is $50 billion of real money.

But let's look at the mechanics.

This is not a block grant. It is not an automatic payment to keep the lights on.

It is a contest.

To get a dime, a state must submit a "detailed rural health transformation plan". They have to hire consultants. They have to draft proposals. They have to prove that their plan will improve "access and quality of care" through "strategic partnerships".

This is grant-writing theater.

The Centers for Medicare & Medicaid Services (CMS) holds the keys. They decide who wins.

And here is the catch.

States cannot use this money to "finance the non-federal share of Medicaid or CHIP".

Translation: You can't use this money to actually pay for healthcare.

You can use it to buy iPads for telemedicine. You can use it to hold seminars on "workforce resilience." You can use it to build a new reception area.

But you cannot use it to pay the doctor's salary. You cannot use it to cover the operating loss from treating poor patients.

It is capital funding in an operating crisis.

It is like giving a starving man a gift card to a furniture store. He doesn't need a sofa. He needs a sandwich.

Now look at what the bill *takes away* to pay for this mirage.

Section 71115 freezes the provider taxes that states use to fund Medicaid. That is the actual operating cash. That is the money that pays the bills *today*.

Section 71113 defunds Essential Community Providers who offer reproductive care. That forces clinics to close.

The bill destroys the foundation of the house, then offers you a coupon for new curtains.

The math is brutal.

The $50 billion is temporary. It expires in 2030.

The cuts to Medicaid are permanent.

The freeze on provider taxes is permanent.

The purge of immigrants from the insurance rolls is permanent.

By the time the "Transformation" money runs out, the landscape will be barren.

The bill calls this "Protecting Rural Hospitals."

In ecology, there is a term for what happens when you remove the water from an ecosystem but plant a few decorative cacti.

It is called desertification.

The "Transformation Program" is not an oasis. It is a mirage.

You can walk toward it. You can write the grant proposals. You can follow the rules.

But when you get there, you will find it is just sand.

And the hospital is still closed.

CITATIONS

SECTION 71401

"Under the program, states may apply for financial allotments to improve the access and quality of care of services in rural areas... States must submit detailed rural health transformation plans..."

SECTION 71115

"The section precludes states that have not expanded Medicaid from increasing the rate of a provider tax beyond that currently in effect in order to qualify for federal matching funds."

SECTION 71113

"This section prohibits federal Medicaid payment... if the provider (1) primarily furnishes family planning services..."

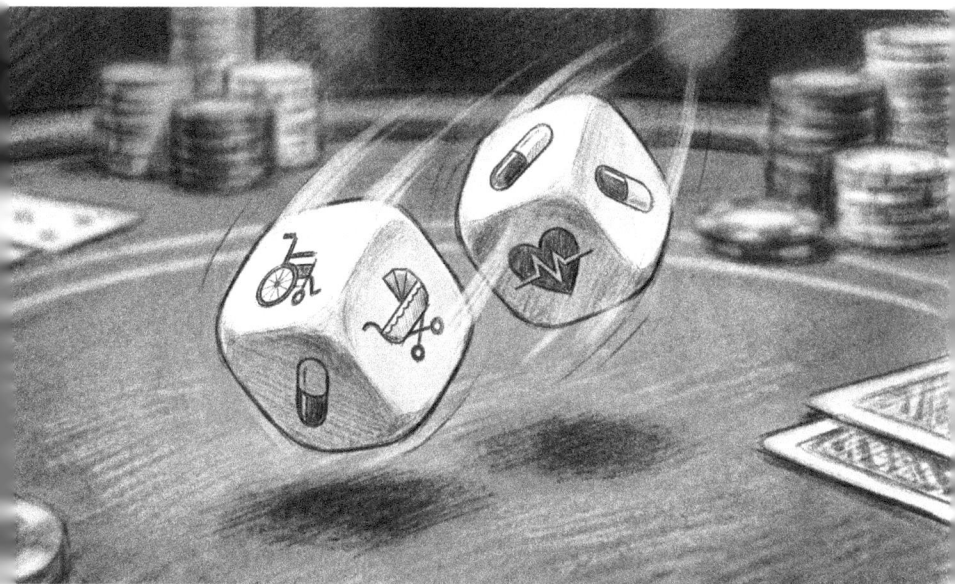

THE MORAL HAZARD

Economists use the term "moral hazard" to describe a situation where someone takes a risk because someone else bears the cost.

If you have insurance, you might drive faster. If you are a bank "too big to fail," you might gamble with depositors' money.

H.R. 1 creates the ultimate moral hazard. It allows politicians to gamble with the healthcare infrastructure, while you pay the price in blood and bone.

The gamble takes two forms. One targets the beginning of life. The other targets the end.

First, the clinics.

Section 71113 is a laser-guided missile. It is designed to look like a ban on abortion funding. It prohibits Medicaid payments to any nonprofit "essential community provider" that primarily furnishes family planning services and offers abortions.

The exceptions are the standard grim trio: rape, incest, or a life-threatening condition.

If a provider crosses this line, they lose everything. They don't just lose funding for the abortion. They lose funding for the pap smear. They lose funding for the breast exam. They lose funding for the contraception that prevents the abortion in the first place.

In a wealthy suburb, this is a political statement. You drive past the defunded clinic to the private OB-GYN down the street.

In rural America, this is a catastrophe.

In many counties, the "family planning" clinic is the *only* clinic. It is the primary care provider for thousands of low-income women. It is where they manage their diabetes. It is where they get their flu shots.

When you defund the clinic to stop abortions, you don't just stop abortions. You stop prenatal care. You stop cancer screenings.

You create a medical vacuum.

The bill authors know this. They don't care. They have health insurance. They have cars. They are insulated from the risk.

That is the moral hazard.

Now look at the nursing homes.

Section 71111 attacks the other end of the spectrum.

In 2024, the government finally admitted a dark truth: nursing homes are understaffed. They issued a rule requiring facilities to have a registered nurse onsite 24 hours a day, 7 days a week.

It seems like a low bar. If you are housing hundreds of sick, frail, elderly people, having *one* nurse in the building at 3:00 AM seems like a minimum safety standard.

H.R. 1 disagrees.

The bill delays this rule. It pushes the implementation date to fiscal year 2035.

That is a ten-year delay.

Think about the cynicism of that date. The average stay in a nursing home is less than three years.

The people in those beds today will be dead by 2035.

The bill essentially says: "We can afford to wait."

It creates a "safe harbor" for the nursing home industry. It protects their profit margins. It spares them the cost of hiring that night-shift nurse.

Who bears the risk?

Your grandmother.

She bears the risk when she falls at 2:00 AM and nobody answers the call button for forty-five minutes. She bears the risk when she develops a bedsore because there weren't enough aides to turn her over.

The politicians get to claim they are "reducing regulatory burdens." They get to say they are "saving the industry."

They are gambling with the safety of the most vulnerable people in the country.

This is not a culture war. A culture war is a debate on cable news.

This is a demolition.

They are dismantling the infrastructure of care for poor women and removing the safety rails for the elderly.

They are doing it because they can. Because the people who suffer—the single mother in the rural clinic, the dementia patient in the understaffed home—cannot donate to a Super PAC.

The bill calls this "Preventing Wasteful Spending".

But there is nothing wasteful about a nurse. There is nothing wasteful about a cancer screening.

The only waste is the time we have lost believing that this bill is about healthcare.

It is about power. And who gets to survive it.

CITATIONS

SECTION 71113

"prohibits federal Medicaid payment... if the provider (1) primarily furnishes family planning services, and (2) performs an abortion..."

SECTION 71111

"This section delays until FY2035 implementation of... Minimum Staffing Standards for Long-Term Care Facilities... that, among other changes, (1) establish minimum staffing standards for nurses in Medicare and Medicaid long-term care facilities..."

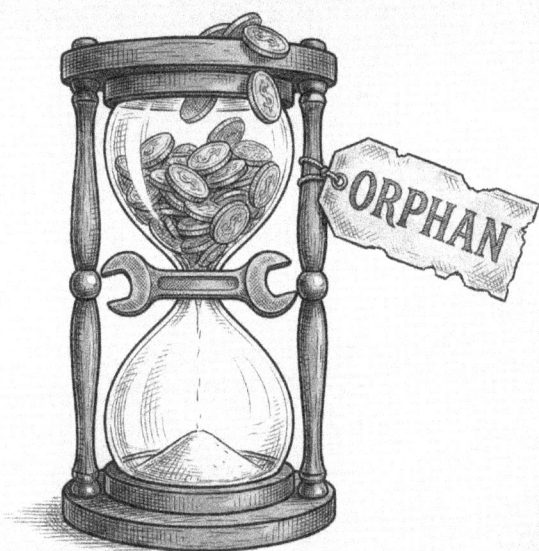

THE RARE DISEASE TRAP

A loophole is not an accident. It is a product feature.

In Washington, the most expensive products are the ones you don't see.

Section 71203 is a multi-billion dollar product. It is sold as compassion. It is engineered as a shield.

Here is the context.

The government finally decided to negotiate drug prices. For decades, Medicare just paid whatever the sticker said. If a pill cost $1,000, Medicare paid $1,000.

The Inflation Reduction Act changed that. It gave Medicare the power to sit at the table. It said, "We will negotiate the price of the biggest, most expensive drugs."

But there was an exception.

They carved out "Orphan Drugs."

These are drugs for rare diseases. Conditions that affect fewer than 200,000 people. The logic was sound. We want companies to invent cures for rare cancers. We don't want to scare them away with price caps.

So the rule was simple: If your drug treats *only one* rare disease, you are safe. No negotiation.

But if you find a second use? If you turn your rare cancer drug into a mass-market blockbuster? The shield drops. You have to negotiate.

H.R. 1 puts the shield back up.

Section 71203 rewrites the rule. It says a drug is exempt even if it treats *more than one* rare disease.

This sounds technical. It is actually a roadmap for price gouging.

Pharmaceutical companies are efficient. They know how to game the system.

They will stop looking for one cure for a big disease. They will look for five cures for five "rare" diseases using the same molecule.

They will stack the indications.

Indication A: Rare stomach cancer. (Exempt). Indication B: Rare throat condition. (Still Exempt). Indication C: Rare blood disorder. (Forever Exempt).

Suddenly, you have a drug that treats 500,000 people. It generates billions in revenue. It is a blockbuster in everything but name.

But under Section 71203, it is legally an "Orphan."

Medicare cannot touch the price.

The bill goes further. It changes the clock.

Usually, a drug becomes eligible for negotiation after it has been on the market for a certain number of years (7 for pills, 11 for biologics).

Section 71203 says that any time spent as an "Orphan" drug *doesn't count* toward that clock.

You could sell a drug for ten years at monopoly prices. Then, you find a mass-market use. The clock should have run out. You should be ready for negotiation.

But this bill pauses the timer. You get to restart the clock.

You get another decade of high prices.

The losers are the seniors.

They are the ones standing at the pharmacy counter. They are the ones in the "donut hole."

They will pay for this loophole with their premiums. They will pay with their deductibles.

The winners are the patent holders.

They just bought themselves immunity from the free market.

They call it the "Rare Disease" exception.

But there is nothing rare about the greed.

CITATIONS

SECTION 71203

"excludes orphan drugs that are approved to treat more than one rare disease or condition from the program... It also excludes any period in which a drug was an orphan drug from market approval calculations."

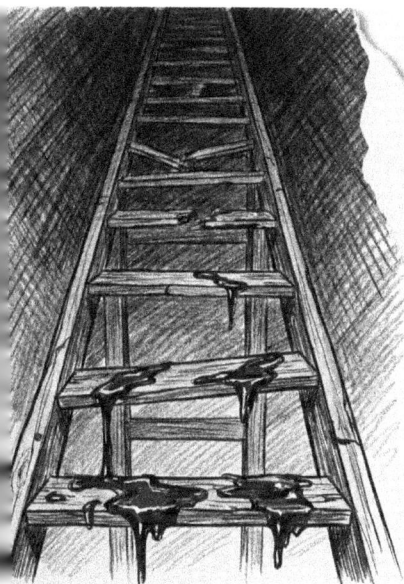

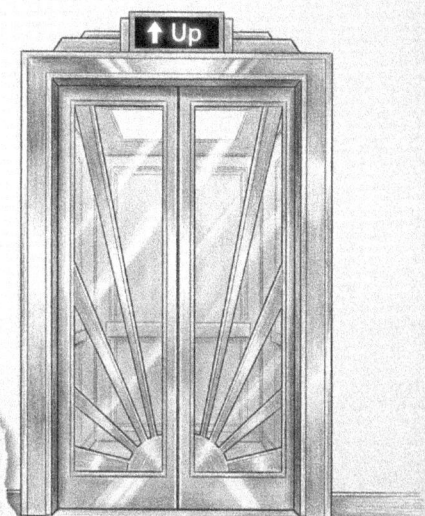

THE SPLIT SCREEN

The genius of H.R. 1 is that it creates two different countries. They occupy the same map. They share the same zip codes. But the people living in them experience a completely different reality.

To understand the bill, you have to watch the split screen.

On the left side of the screen, we have the Winners. On the right side, we have the Losers.

Let's turn on the audio.

Screen Left: The Estate of Grace

Life is good here.

You are wealthy. You have assets. And the government just gave you a permanent gift.

Section 70106 doubles the exemption for the Estate Tax. You can now pass down $15 million tax-free. That is a dynasty builder.

Your business is booming. Section 70301 makes "bonus depreciation" permanent. You buy a corporate jet. You write off the entire cost immediately. You don't wait years to get your tax break. You get it today.

You want to drill for oil? The government is practically handing you the keys to the Arctic National Wildlife Refuge. They are slashing your royalty rates. They are reinstating noncompetitive leasing.

You have a kid? The government opens a "Trump Account" for them. They deposit $1,000 of federal money just because your child was born. You can stuff another $5,000 a year into it, tax-advantaged.

Compound interest is your best friend.

Screen Right: The Hunger Freeze

Life is harder here.

You are hungry. You rely on SNAP (food stamps) to feed your family.

Section 10101 freezes your reality.

It prohibits the USDA from updating the "Thrifty Food Plan" based on what food actually costs. It tethers the benefit to a generic inflation index.

If the price of healthy food spikes, the formula doesn't care. The math ignores the price of broccoli. It ignores the price of meat.

Your buying power shrinks every year.

You are an immigrant. You followed the rules. You were granted asylum because your life was in danger.

Section 71109 says you are no longer welcome on Medicaid. Section 10108 kicks you off SNAP.

You are a "legal" resident. You have papers. But you aren't a citizen yet.

The safety net dissolves.

You are unemployed. You are looking for work.

Section 71119 demands you clock 80 hours of activity a month just to see a doctor.

You spend your days chasing paperwork. You spend your nights worrying about the "recapture" letter from the IRS that says you owe $5,000 for your health insurance subsidy.

The Transfer

Now look at the middle of the screen.

This is where the magic trick happens.

The bill claims to "reduce the deficit." It claims to be about "fiscal responsibility."

But the money is moving.

It moves from the pockets of the asylum seeker to the pockets of the oil executive.

It moves from the rural hospital losing its provider tax funding to the corporate shareholder enjoying a lower tax rate.

It moves from the "Thrifty Food Plan" to the "Trump Account".

This is not savings. This is extraction.

The bill extracts stability from the poor to subsidize risk for the rich.

It takes the certainty of a meal away from a child. It gives the certainty of a tax cut to a millionaire.

Section 70501 and 70502 repeal the tax credits for clean vehicles. That money is gone.

Where did it go?

It went to Section 50403. That section pours money into "energy infrastructure reinvestment" but specifically *removes* financing for products that reduce greenhouse gas emissions.

It pays to pollute.

The Verdict

The split screen resolves into a single image.

It is a picture of a ladder.

H.R. 1 greases the rungs at the bottom. It makes it harder to climb. It makes it easier to slip.

If you fall, there is no net.

But at the top?

At the top, they are building an elevator.

CITATIONS

SECTION 70106

"This section increases the base estate tax... exemption amount after 2025 to $15 million..."

SECTION 70301

"This section permanently extends 100% bonus depreciation for property acquired and placed into service... on or after January 19, 2025."

SECTION 70204

"This section establishes a new type of tax-advantaged account, called a Trump account... authorizes a one-time federal government deposit of $1,000 into a Trump account..."

SECTION 10101

"This section prohibits USDA from increasing the cost of the Thrifty Food Plan (TFP) based on a reevaluation of the contents of the TFP..."

SECTION 71109

"Current law authorizes federal payment with respect to additional categories of individuals, including refugees... The section excludes these individuals from eligibility."

SECTION 71119

"individuals... must demonstrate compliance... on a monthly basis, (1) work at least 80 hours..."

SECTIONS 70501 & 70502

"This section terminates the previously-owned clean vehicle tax credit... This section terminates the clean vehicle tax credit."

SECTION 50403

"revises the types of projects eligible for energy infrastructure re-investment financing. In particular, this financing is eliminated for projects that avoid or reduce air pollutants or greenhouse gas (GHG) emissions."

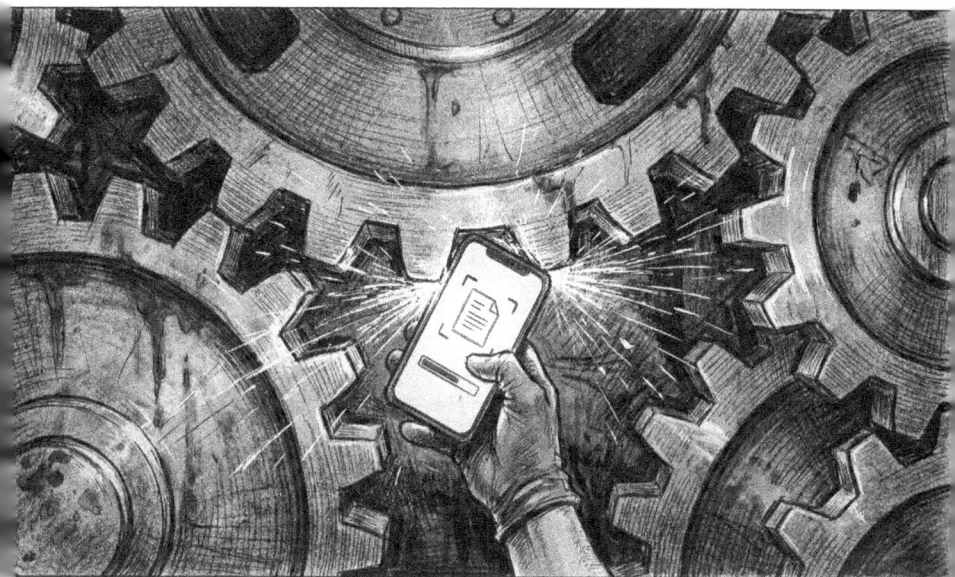

CONCLUSION:
HOW TO SURVIVE THE MACHINE

The ink is dry.

The President signed it on July 4th. There were fireworks. There were speeches about freedom.

While the sky exploded, the gears of H.R. 1 started to turn.

You cannot stop it now. The bill is law. The new debt limit is set. The tax cuts are permanent. The work requirements are live.

You are inside the machine.

The machine is not evil. It is indifferent. It is an algorithm designed to save money by identifying friction points and applying pressure.

If you break, it saves a dollar.

So the goal is simple. Do not break.

You need a strategy. You need a defense manual for the next ten years.

Rule 1: Digitize or Die.

The bill relies on paper. It relies on the lost letter. It relies on the form that gets stuck in the mailroom.

Do not trust the mail.

Section 71107 demands you verify your life every six months. If you miss a deadline, you are a ghost.

Buy a scanner. Or use your phone. Every pay stub. Every utility bill. Every tax return. Scan it the second you touch it. Upload it to the cloud.

When the state says "We never received your proof of community service," you don't argue. You email the PDF. You fax the screenshot. You overwhelm their silence with data.

Be paranoid. The "Death Master File" is looking for a reason to delete you. Do not give it one.

Rule 2: Dodge the Clawback.

The IRS is now a debt collector for your health insurance.

Section 71305 removed the cap. If you underestimate your income, they will take everything back.

Do not guess.

If you are a freelancer, assume you will have a good year. Estimate high. It will make your monthly premium more expensive. It will hurt.

But it is better to pay $50 more a month now than to owe the IRS $8,000 next April.

Treat your tax credit like a loan shark. Pay it respect. Or it will break your legs.

Rule 3: Avoid the Bronze Trap.

They will tempt you with low premiums. They will show you a "Catastrophic" plan that costs $20 a month. They will tell you to put money in an HSA.

Do not take the bait.

Unless you have $10,000 sitting in a bank account right now, that plan is not insurance. It is a bankruptcy filing waiting to happen.

If you get sick on a Bronze plan, you are alone. You are on the hook for the first $9,000.

Buy the Silver plan if you can. Eat rice and beans if you have to. The "savings" on the premium are a mirage.

Rule 4: Build a Parallel Network.

The rural hospital is closing. The "Transformation Fund" is just buying them new iPads.

The clinic down the road lost its funding because of Section 71113.

You cannot rely on the infrastructure. It is being liquidated.

Find the community health center. Find the charity care network. Know where they are before you have the chest pain.

If you have a car, keep it running. You might need to drive two counties over to give birth. The local delivery room is gone.

The Final Ghost

This book started with a warning about ghosts.

The 10 million people who will vanish from the rolls.

The machine wants you to be one of them. It wants you to get tired. It wants you to look at the 80-hour work requirement form and say "It's too much."

It wants you to fade.

Do not fade.

The "One Big Beautiful Bill Act" is a test. It is testing how much friction you can endure.

It pushes. You have to push back.

They built a casino where the house always wins. They rigged the wheel. They marked the cards.

But you are still at the table.

Check your paperwork. Watch your income. Guard your status.

Survive.

CITATIONS

SECTION 71107

"requires state Medicaid programs to redetermine every six months... the eligibility of individuals who are enrolled in Medicaid as part of the Medicaid expansion population..."

SECTION 71305

"eliminates the limit on the recapture of excess advance payments of the premium tax credit and, accordingly, allows the full amount of any such excess payments to be recaptured."

SECTION 71113

"prohibits federal Medicaid payment... if the provider (1) primarily furnishes family planning services..."

www.ingramcontent.com/pod-product-compliance
Lightning Source LLC
Chambersburg PA
CBHW020007290326
41935CB00007B/335